YOUR KNOWLEDGE HAS VALUE

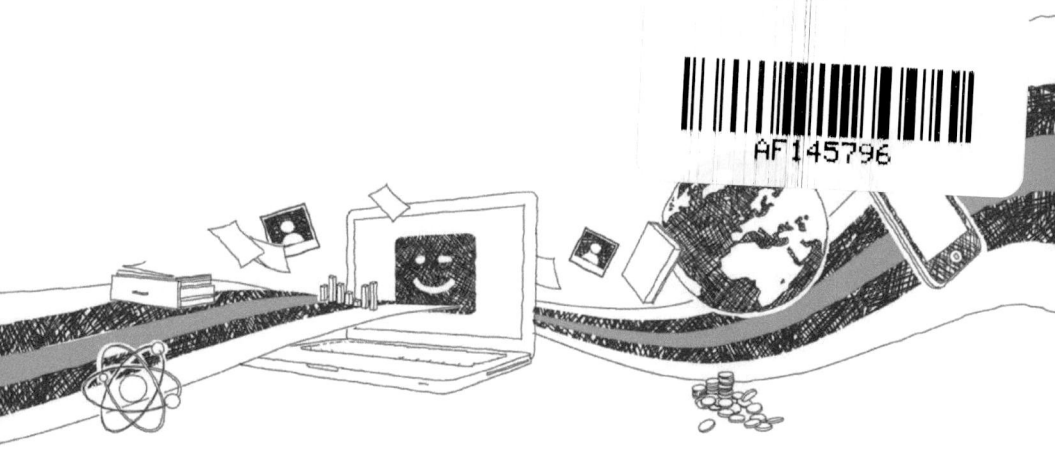

- We will publish your bachelor's and
  master's thesis, essays and papers

- Your own eBook and book -
  sold worldwide in all relevant shops

- Earn money with each sale

Upload your text at www.GRIN.com
and publish for free

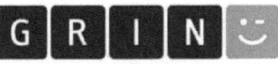

Bibliographic information published by the German National Library:

The German National Library lists this publication in the National Bibliography; detailed bibliographic data are available on the Internet at http://dnb.dnb.de .

Imprint:

Copyright © 2016 GRIN Verlag
Print and binding: Books on Demand GmbH, Norderstedt Germany
ISBN: 9783668760851

This book at GRIN:

https://www.grin.com/document/432528

Natascha Dremov

Can the German health care system be adapted to India?

GRIN Verlag

GRIN - Your knowledge has value

Since its foundation in 1998, GRIN has specialized in publishing academic texts by students, college teachers and other academics as e-book and printed book. The website www.grin.com is an ideal platform for presenting term papers, final papers, scientific essays, dissertations and specialist books.

Visit us on the internet:

http://www.grin.com/

http://www.facebook.com/grincom

http://www.twitter.com/grin_com

Can the German health care system be adapted to India?

Natascha Dremov, 11Pp
Schuljahr 2015/16
Abgabetermin 09.05.2016

Table of Contents

1 Introduction

The health care of every country is utterly significant for the well-being of every citizen. Gandhi recognized the importance of health. And he was right. Health has to be achievable for every person. A good health care system provides help when needed and moreover also often bears the costs of the treatment. When a good system is given, the life expectancy increases, because many diseases are recognized earlier if a doctor is visited. With the growth of the population the significance of the health sector increases continuously. [2]

Even when no medical treatment is needed, many people feel safer when they have the guarantee to get one if it is required. This gives a secure feeling to the inhabitants of the country. It makes the citizens believe in their own government. Although a well-organized health care system has so many advantages for all of the population, sadly most of the Indians do not have medical insurance at all.[3]

Good health care needs to be affordable and available for every single inhabitant of a country. Therefore you need proper infrastructure and a very thorough organization. In my thesis paper I will explain the current situation in medical care in India and the problems connected with it. I will list the reasons that led to this state and picture their influence on India. After that, I want to shortly summarize the problem India has with its healthcare system. As a next step, I will be explaining the German healthcare system with the German health insurances. In addition I want to list some advantages and disadvantages the German insurance system has. In the next paragraphs I will check whether the German system is adaptable to India to improve the Indian health care situation. For that two different projects in India will be explained to illustrate the attempt to improve the system. The answer whether the German health care system would be possible in India will be stated in the last part of the paper, the conclusion.

2 The Indian health care system

2.1 Private health care

India´s medical care is full of contrasts. If you are wealthy enough, you can get access to the best clinics around the world. India´s leading universities spawn some of the best medics. Furthermore through the last few decades a lot of modern, western hospitals were

---

[1] http://www.mkgandhi.org/articles/g_health.htm (last visited on 01.05.16)
[2] http://www.vsfs.cz/prilohy/konference/1_ws_3_1_theodopulos.doc (last visited on 08.04.16)
[3] http://www.brandeins.de/wissen/hilfe/hilfe-das-pharmamagazin/wie-gehts-indien/ (last visited on 08.04.16)

built in India. These hospitals are equipped with latest technologies. Unfortunately about eight out of ten people are not rich enough to afford treatments in corporations like "Apollo" or "Fortis", the biggest groups of healthcare in India.[4]

Nevertheless it is estimated that private sector hospitals are responsible for around 70% of the medical care in urban areas as most of the people avoid public clinics. Whereas owing to bad access in rural areas, people outside big cities depend more on public health care.[5]

2.2 Public health care

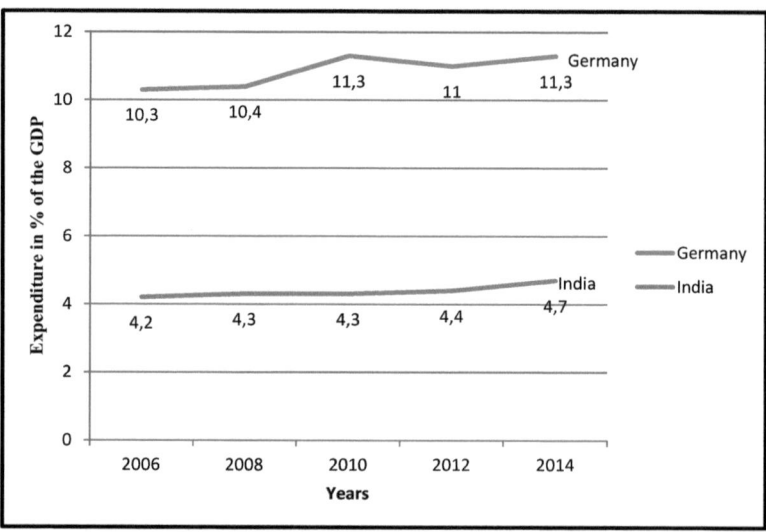

Fig. 1: Health expenditure, total (% of GDP) (data based on
http://data.worldbank.org/indicator/SH.XPD.TOTL.ZS/countries/1W-IN-DE?display=graph)

If you compare India's expenditure on health care, you will probably be very surprised. In comparison to other countries it is very low. India's expenditure is about 4.7% of the GDP Germany's is about 11.3%.(Fig. 1).[6] Germany is representative for many European countries like Switzerland, the Netherlands and France. India's expenses on the other hand serve to illustrate a similar situation in some African developing countries just as several Asian countries. The slight increase in India's expenditure during the last ten years could be

[4] http://www.thenational.ae/business/economy/indians-faced-with-overcrowded-public-hospitals-turn-to-private-clinics#full (last visited on 08.04.16)
[5] http://dhsprogram.com/pubs/pdf/FRIND3/FRIND3-Vol1AndVol2.pdf (last visited on 08.04.16)
[6] http://data.worldbank.org/indicator/SH.XPD.TOTL.ZS?order=wbapi_data_value_2013+wbapi_data_value+wbapi_data_value-last&sort=desc (last visited on 07.05.16)

explained by several projects and missions India launched. The projects should lead to an improved health care system. In later parts of my thesis paper some of these missions will be explained.

Due to bad infrastructure and mostly poor areas, private clinics are rarely found in rural India. As mentioned before, here usually people depend on public hospitals. [7]

This results in a catastrophic situation in government clinics. The part of the citizens who lives below poverty line has free access to public health care. Though this fact seems rather helpful for poor people, rural hospitals mostly offer just a very low quality of treatments. In addition the hospitals are often too crowded, there is insufficient space for every individual and waiting times are so long that you rarely get the treatment or operation in time.[5]

2.3 Reasons for the current state

There are countless reasons for the current situation in India. The following points, "poverty, population and illiteracy" are not the only ones. More reasons could be wrongly set priorities from the government in the past or not estimated effects of decisions the government made. Nevertheless the following three arguments are crucial for the development of the country. Even though the three reasons all depend on each other and determine each other, every single one of them has its own aftermaths.

2.3.1 Poverty

The international poverty line is defined on $ 1,25 income per day. An estimated third of India's population is living below this line.[8] Some even think that more people fall below the poverty line because $ 1,25 are not enough to afford proper shelter and enough food, not to mention proper conditions in hygiene and access to decent toilets.[9]

There are other groups of inhabitants, who are not even mentioned in the poverty count. Some of the poorest people are the so-called "untouchables". They are not counted, because they live at the bottom of society and are not accepted.[10]

As already said, poverty has lots of effects on health. Not being able to afford decent shelter means being exposed to the environment and all its circumstances. Rain, storm, drought and heat affect the human body. Heat strokes, heart strokes and dehydration are only some of the effects.

---

[7] https://en.wikipedia.org/wiki/Healthcare_in_India (last visited on 01.05.16)
[8] http://www.mapsofindia.com/my-india/india/overpopulation-in-india-causes-effects-and-how-to-control-it (last visited on 10.04.16)
[9] http://www.poverties.org/poverty-in-india.html (last visited on 08.04.16)
[10] http://www.poverties.org/poverty-in-india.html (last visited on 08.04.16)

Further, big parts of Indian population are malnourished because they cannot afford decent, nutritious food. As a result, children and adolescents develop slowly or even die at a very young age. 98 out of 1000 children die before their fifth birthday. [11]

In addition more than 2/3 of all people in India are not able to go to a hygienic toilet or lavatories. Consequently, bacteria colonies have the chance to grow rapidly. Not being able to wash oneself, diseases will spread even faster.[10]

On average, an Indian adult has an income of less than $120 per month.[12] In comparison, a cheap surgical operation in India costs about $500. This may seem cheap for European standards but is rather expensive for a normal local worker.[13]

2.3.2 Population

India has a very high population in comparison to other countries. With it's 1.2 billion inhabitants it is the country with the second largest population after China. Nevertheless this is not as important as the population density. In Indian big cities it is multiple times higher than in big cities in Germany. For instance Berlin has a population density of 3.900 per km^2. This seems like nothing in comparison to the density in Mumbai, the biggest city in India. Mumbai has a density of 20.000 per km^2. The huge number of people especially in metropolises like Mumbai has a lot of aftermaths, not only on the health care situation.[14] [15]

High population growth in India is also one of the reasons for growing resource use. The growth rate 2013 was 1.25%. The fertility rate is almost 70 % higher than in Germany. [16] Increasing population needs a growing number of resources like water or food, better infrastructure, more area for living and many more things. That can be utterly expensive for a country. [17]

One of the effects the overpopulation has in India is the bad water supply and waste disposal. This leads to a catastrophic situation in hygiene. When clean water is not available, people cannot drink as much as they need. To add, they do not get the opportunity to wash themselves or their hands. As a consequence bacteria can get in uncleaned wounds, or viruses and germs can get into the body through the mouth while eating. This can cause infected wounds, gastritis and almost any contagious disease.

---

[11] http://www.patengemeinschaft.de/seiten/indien/land.html (last visited on 08.04.16)
[12] http://durchschnittseinkommen.net/durchschnittseinkommen-indien/ (last visited on 2904.16)
[13] http://www.welt.de/gesundheit/article116481982/Klinik-bietet-Herz-Operationen-fuer-1390-Euro-an.html (last visited on 10.04.16)
[14] https://de.wikipedia.org/wiki/Berlin (last visited on 07.05.16)
[15] https://de.wikipedia.org/wiki/Mumbai (last visited on 07.05.16)
[16] https://en.wikipedia.org/wiki/Demographics_of_India (last visited on 01.05.16)
[17] http://www.mapsofindia.com/my-india/india/overpopulation-in-india-causes-effects-and-how-to-control-it (last visited on 10.04.16)

The government is trying to improve the situation in India by controlling growth of inhabitants by eliminating or lessen the reasons for overpopulation. Illiteracy, which is another point in my thesis paper, is hoped to be decreased by sex education and spreading awareness. This would not only help decreasing birth rate but also hinder sexually transmitted diseases to spread.[18]

2.3.3   Illiteracy

Literacy is simply known as the ability to read and write. Consequently illiteracy is not being able to do so. In the following paragraphs I will not focus on the ability to read, but rather on all the things connected to it. Literacy also can mean to be aware of consequences that actions have and being aware of how illnesses and STDs spread. Furthermore it can mean going to school, understanding, interpreting and also being able to use common sense to question specific issues.

India's illiterate population is known to be the largest in the world. Nearly 300 million adults in India cannot write nor read. This cannot just cause a lower income or even unemployment. It can also have impacts on the health of the individual. As mentioned before, illiterate adults often are not aware of their illnesses or diseases. Some misuse medication, some do not understand the importance of medical care. Therefore many underestimate the significance of their health.[19]

There are particular tribal populations who have their very own way of dealing with diseases. They do not see an illness as a biological effect of germs but rather as some kind of punishment or lesson for the person. As a result they have their own cures and methods to heal. An example for this is Ayurveda. It's a traditional, plant-based system of medicine from India.[20] Although there are people who believe that Ayurvedic medicine can cure almost any disease, on the contrary there is also lot's of criticism. Researchers from the University Of Pennsylvania School Of Medicine tested the effectiveness of some Ayurvedic methods. They claim that the tested treatments had no effect at all. [21]

Taking everything into account, illiteracy and the resulting wrong methods of dealing with illnesses cause unwanted effects on health. Increasing literacy rate and making people aware of risks would help to diagnose and treat diseases before they become a real danger. It follows that this would relieve hospitals, increase life expectancy and help to eliminate illnesses.

---

[18] http://www.mapsofindia.com/my-india/india/overpopulation-in-india-causes-effects-and-how-to-control-it (last visited on 10.04.16)
[19] https://www.fondationalphabetisation.org/en/foundation/causes-of-illiteracy/consequences-of-illiteracy/ (last visited on 17.04.16)
[20] https://mygov.in/sites/default/files/user_comments/Current_Health.pdf (last visited on 17.0416)
[21] http://www.skeptic.com/eskeptic/13-10-09/#note12 (last visited on17.04.16)

2.4 The Problem

On the whole you can say that the health care system only works well for those who can afford it. Latest technologies and well-educated doctors are available only for the wealthy.

In contrast to private clinics stand government hospitals. In view of the low expenditures on health care from the government in the past years, an undeniably poor situation resulted. Government hospitals seem to be available for everyone but nevertheless they solely offer an inferior treatment.

3 The German health care system

3.1 Basic information

The probably most important difference between German and Indian health care is the fact that Germany has a compulsory health insurance for everybody. Every citizen has to have Statutory Health Insurance. Those, who earn enough money, can even conclude Private Health Insurance. All the money is collected by health care funds and will be paid off when needed. [22] [23]

3.2 Statutory Health Insurance

Employees and employers pay health insurance monthly. The amount of dues is dependent on the income of the person. Generally 14,6% of the gross wage has to be paid to the insurance. With Statutory Health Insurance family members are insured automatically. [24]

Statutory Health Insurance is based on the principle of solidarity. This means that medical coverage will be provided mainly through money collected by the funds. Additional expenses are brought up by taxes, which are paid by all of the inhabitants.[25] As a result, every insured citizen pays for others. In return in case of illness he has the right on a proper treatment, paid by healthy insured inhabitants. [26]

The majority of hospitals, dental clinics and for example physical therapists are paid from the Statutory Health Insurance. It is not necessary to raise your own money in case of illness. [27]

---

[22] https://en.wikipedia.org/wiki/Healthcare_in_Germany (last visited on 07.05.16)
[23] https://www.gesundheitsinformation.de/das-deutsche-gesundheitssystem.2698.de.html?part=einleitung-co (last visited on 07.05.16)
[24] http://www.bmg.bund.de/themen/krankenversicherung/finanzierung/finanzierungsgrundlagen-der-gesetzlichen-krankenversicherung.html (last visited on 07.05.16)
[25] https://www.gesundheitsinformation.de/das-deutsche-gesundheitssystem.2698.de.html?part=einleitung-co (last visited on 07.05.16)
[26] https://www.justlanded.com/deutsch/Deutschland/Artikel/Gesundheit/Die-2-Arten-der-Krankenversicherung (last visited on 07.05.16)
[27] https://www.gesundheitsinformation.de/das-deutsche-gesundheitssystem.2698.de.html?part=einleitung-co (last visited on 07.05.16)

With Insurance important medications are provided freely or reduced in price. In addition, hospitalization and medical or dental treatment is always guaranteed. Furthermore, Statutory Insurance also pays for disease prevention. This means for instance vaccination and cancer check-ups. Besides, insured people always have the right to get screenings and medical check-ups. Methods for early diagnosis of diseases are also provided. [28]

3.3 Private Health Insurance

Those who earn enough money can conclude Private Health Insurance. The main difference between Statutory and Private Health insurance is that Private Health insurance is based on another principle, the principle of individuality. This means that every insured person provides money for its own disease risk. For that the costs will be adjusted individually dependent on health situation, age and extent of the Insurance services.[29]

Germans with Private Health Insurance sometimes have advantages like being preferred when waiting for doctors or being able to choose their services freely. In addition, money for not utilized treatments will be paid back. [30]

On the other hand, private insurance has some downsides to it. For example family members have to pay a reduced due, instead of being included in the insurance. Fees also could climb very high in case of severe diseases. Besides, private insurance always asks you to pay your medical bills yourself first, before later restoring the costs.[31]

3.4 Other types of insurances for health

There are even more types of insurances like the accident insurance, which prevents work accidents and helps injured people to step by step get back to work.[32]

Furthermore there is a long term care insurance which provides nursing when the person is dependent on care. It even covers the case if a person is suffering from dementia or is disabled physically or mentally. This insurance makes sure that assistance is given several hours per day. [33]

---

[28] http://www.deutsche-sozialversicherung.de/de/krankenversicherung/leistungen.html (last visited on 07.05.16)
[29] https://www.justlanded.com/deutsch/Deutschland/Artikel/Gesundheit/Die-2-Arten-der-Krankenversicherung (last visited on 07.05.16)
[30] https://www.private-krankenversicherungen-testsieger.de/private-krankenversicherung-vorteile-und-nachteile/ (last visited on 07.05.16)
[31] https://www.private-krankenversicherungen-testsieger.de/private-krankenversicherung-vorteile-und-nachteile/ (last visited on 07.05.16)
[32] https://de.wikipedia.org/wiki/Gesetzliche_Unfallversicherung_in_Deutschland (last visited on 07.05.16)
[33] https://en.wikipedia.org/wiki/Long-term_care_insurance_in_Germany (last visited on 07.05.16)

3.5 Conclusion

You can safely say that having compulsory health insurance for every inhabitant has many advantages. In case of sickness people do not have to worry about saving money for their medical fees. Moreover surgery and care is always guaranteed.

On the contrary, in many countries people with lower income cannot afford insurance. Sometimes, insurance in other countries like India or the USA even has limited doctor visits. [34] Further it can be very expensive for the government to bring up additional budget from taxes, if the health funds cannot collect sufficient money. In addition it is also rather costly for the whole country to build hospitals where required and improve infrastructure to ensure everyone has access to medical treatment.

4 German system adapted to India

Germany seems to have an utterly well-organized system, where help, care, prescription drugs or surgery is guaranteed when needed. This method is used in many European countries. India saw its crisis several years ago and started projects to improve the situation and tried to offer everybody the care they needed, similar as in European countries. Since average income in India is very low and big parts of the population live below the international poverty line, the government and the provinces have to raise the incidental costs themselves. In the following paragraphs I will explain how India attempts to solve the difficult situation through two different projects. In the next steps I want to analyze whether such a system is even possible and whether it has a future in India. Therefore I will weigh all chances the projects have and all arising difficulties.

4.1 RSBY - Rashtriya Swasthya Bima Yojana

The RSBY is an Indian mission, launched in 2008. Rashtriya Swasthya Bima Yojana, the Indian name for this project can be translated to National Health Insurance Program. The main idea of it is to cover a specific amount of the medical fees for the poorest parts of the population. At first it was supposed to cover all people below poverty line. However, it was later extended for other groups like unorganized mine workers, domestic workers, rickshaw pullers and many others. [35]

RSBY shall pay for hospitalization costs up to 30.000 Rs which is equal to 400 €. Furthermore even transportation expenses to the hospitals will be paid up to a certain amount. [36]

---

[34] http://patch.com/pennsylvania/foresthills-regentsquare/bp--pros-cons-to-having-health-insurance-3935cfce (last visited on 24.04.16)
[35] http://www.rsby.gov.in/about_rsby.aspx (last visited on 24.04.16)
[36] http://www.rsby.gov.in/about_rsby.aspx (last visited on 24.04.16)

For registering a person only needs to give their fingerprint and a charge of 30 Rs, which is less than half a Euro. The rest of the expenses are covered by central and state government. Then the person will be given a small card, their own Smart Card, with which up to four additional family members can be insured, too. [37]

Today more than 12.000 hospitals are cooperating with this program. 33 Million households already are in possession of the Smart Card. Nevertheless it is estimated that only one third of the population below poverty line has this card. [38] [39]

The whole program was developed by both Indian and German information technologists. While Germany by now has a health insurance for everybody, the system with the Smart Card is new. India can learn from Germany, by offering their poorer inhabitants health care. On the contrary German developers are thinking about introducing a Smart card, too, to improve the German Health Insurance Card. In Germany this system could also be helping local administration, for instance by providing lower-income households subsidization.[40]

4.2 NHAM - National Health Assurance Mission

A second mission was started in 2015 - The National Health Assurance Mission. It is supposed to cover the entire population. This fact stands in contrast to the RSBY, which only covers the poor parts of the population. However, NHAM should be linked to RSBY, so people below poverty line get their insurance for free, whereas others have to pay only little money. [41]

By 2019 the whole population shall be covered by NHAM. In the past years expenses on health were mostly covered out of the pocket. This is hoped to be reduced in the following years and replaced by coverage by the insurance. [42]

Under the NHAM, states are financially supported to improve their health care and offer some free treatments for the population. The services include free immunization against several diseases and free treatments for Malaria or Tuberculosis. Moreover, there are some initiatives which ensure pregnant women to have a free delivery and health screening for the

---

[37] https://www.giz.de/de/downloads/giz2013-de-akzente01-krankenversicherungsprogramm-indien.pdf (last visited on 24.04.16)
[38] https://www.giz.de/de/downloads/giz2013-de-akzente01-krankenversicherungsprogramm-indien.pdf (last visited on 24.04.16)
[39] https://en.wikipedia.org/wiki/Rashtriya_Swasthya_Bima_Yojana (last visited on 24.04.16)
[40] https://www.giz.de/de/downloads/giz2013-de-akzente01-krankenversicherungsprogramm-indien.pdf (last visited on 24.04.16)
[41] http://www.fantasticfundas.com/2015/07/national-health-assurance-mission-nham.html (last visited on 24.04.16)
[42] http://pib.nic.in/newsite/PrintRelease.aspx?relid=106608 (last visited on 24.04.16)

child.[43] 2015 The expected costs for this program were $ 18,5 billion for the following five years. The mission was delayed 2015 due to the high costs.[44]

4.3 Chances

A similar system as in Germany and Europe has many opportunities and chances. It provides ambulatory treatment, hospitalization and care for those in need. This means that a hospital can be visited whenever required. In addition the transportation costs are lessened through the help by RSBY.

One of the great opportunities is the use of the Smart Card, as in the RSBY. Not only is it efficient and effective for a whole family, it has also a very strong psychological effect. In European countries most of the population has a safe feeling, through knowing that insurance will always be provided. This security can now also be given to the poor population.

4.4 Difficulties

Firstly, one big difficulty is obviously the very high price for the government. Many people in India are poor, so they cannot afford insurance themselves. Consequently, the majority of costs have to be covered by the central government and the state governments.

Secondly, access to infrastructure has to be provided. Roads and ways of transport have to be improved, if proper supply wants to be guaranteed. The origin of India's infrastructure is still from British colonization. Most of the railroads are still working but they are not sufficient for the whole population. In conclusion India has to spend a lot of money if India wants to offer all inhabitants enough proper transportation methods. As a result, people in rural areas get a connection to hospitals and doctors. [45]

Thirdly, there is another problem, which has to be solved if India wants its health care system to work. It is the implementation of the programs like NHAM or RSBY. In 2015 the health ministry in New Delhi found out that some states were not using their budget for health legally. As a solution committees were set up by the government to control the proper implementation of the money and the health care missions.[46]

---

[43] http://pib.nic.in/newsite/PrintRelease.aspx?relid=106608 (last visited on 24.04.16)
[44] http://in.reuters.com/article/india-health-idINKBN0MM2UT20150327 (last visited on 24.04.16)
[45] https://www.fmglobal-touchpoints.de/risiken-nutzen/laenderreport-indien/ (last visited on 06.05.16)
[46] http://economictimes.indiatimes.com/news/politics-and-nation/Centre-pulls-up-states-for-poor-implementation-of-National-Rural-Health-Mission/articleshow/50320802.cms (last visited 06.05.16)

5 Conclusion

The German compulsory health care system is based on payments that every employee and their employers pay monthly. For this kind of regulation a country needs employees who have an employment agreement or some kind of data that confirms the labor. Only 10% of all employed people in India have some kind of employment agreement. The rest works illegally and without contract. In conclusion one can say that the German health care system could not be transferred to India. [47]

In addition, India's average income is already so low that most of the simple workers cannot do without every single Rupee. A monthly payment would be almost impossible for normal employees and poor, unemployed inhabitants. Private health insurance bills would be even harder to pay.

To sum up, the German or European health care system is too expensive and nearly impossible in India. Only a tiny fraction of employees has an employment contract and moreover workers wages are too low. Paying dues to a health fund would be way too costly for the average worker. Besides, infrastructure first has to be expanded and improved to guarantee access to hospitals in rural areas.

Nevertheless Gandhi was right as to say that health is most important to every person. India saw the need of proper medical coverage. To solve this situation, India launched some projects to ensure health care to rural and poorer inhabitants. With these projects citizens do not have to pay medical fees themselves. This is a very effective way to start providing care and hospitalization. To conclude, you can say that India is on a good way to improve its health situation.

---

[47] http://durchschnittseinkommen.net/durchschnittseinkommen-indien/ (last visited on 06.05.16)

6 Bibliography

6.1 Printed sources

- Da Cruz, Patrick / Dr. Capallo, Stephan (eds.): *Gesundheitsmegamarkt Indien.* Wiesbaden: Gabler 2008.
- Garrett, Laurie: *Das Ende der Gesundheit: Bericht über die medizinische Lage der Welt.* Berlin: Siedler Verlag 2001.
- Panagariya, Arvind: *India: The emerging giant.* New York: Oxford University Press, Inc. 2008.

6.2 Digital sources

- http://data.worldbank.org/indicator/SH.XPD.TOTL.ZS?order=wbapi_data_value_2013 +wbapi_data_value+wbapi_data_value-last&sort=desc. The world bank: Health expenditure, total (% of GDP). (Withdrawal from the internet: 07.05.16)

- http://dhsprogram.com/pubs/pdf/FRIND3/FRIND3-Vol1AndVol2.pdf. Ministry of Health and Family Welfare Government of India: National Family Health Survey. Publication: 2007. (Withdrawal from the internet: 08.04.16)

- http://durchschnittseinkommen.net/durchschnittseinkommen-indien/. Durchschnittseinkommen In Indien. (Withdrawal from the Internet: 29.04.16)

- http://economictimes.indiatimes.com/news/politics-and-nation/Centre-pulls-up-states-for-poor-implementation-of-National-Rural-Health-Mission/articleshow/50320802.cms. Sushmi Dey: Centre pulls up states for poor implementation of National Rural Health Mission. Publication: 25.12.15. (Withdrawal from the internet: 06.05.17)

- http://in.reuters.com/article/india-health-idINKBN0MM2UT20150327. Aditya Kalra: Exclusive: Modi govt puts brakes on India's universal health plan. Publication: 27.03.15. (Withdrawal from the internet: 24.04.16)

- http://patch.com/pennsylvania/foresthills-regentsquare/bp--pros-cons-to-having-health-insurance-3935cfce. Erika Bogden: Pros & Cons to having Health Insurance. Publication: 05.11.12. (Withdrawal from the internet: 24.04.16)

- http://pib.nic.in/newsite/PrintRelease.aspx?relid=106608. Government of India: Rolling out of National Health Assurance Mission. Publication: 15.07.14. (Withdrawal from the internet: 24.04.16)

- http://www.bmg.bund.de/themen/krankenversicherung/finanzierung/finanzierungsgrundlagen-der-gesetzlichen-krankenversicherung.html. Bundesministerium für Gesundheit: Finanzierungsgrundlagen der gesetzlichen Krankenversicherung.(Withdrawal from the internet: 07.05.16)

- http://www.brandeins.de/wissen/hilfe/hilfe-das-pharmamagazin/wie-gehts-indien/. Gerhard Waldherr: Indien. (Withdrawal from the internet: 08.04.16)

- http://www.deutsche-sozialversicherung.de/de/krankenversicherung/leistungen.html. Deutsche Sozialversicherung Europavertretung: Leistungen. (Withdrawal from the internet: 07.05.16)

- http://www.fantasticfundas.com/2015/07/national-health-assurance-mission-nham.html. Fantastic Fundas: National Health Assurance Mission (NHAM). (Withdrawal from the internet: 24.04.16)

- http://www.mapsofindia.com/my-india/india/overpopulation-in-india-causes-effects-and-how-to-control-it. Rumani Saikia Phukan: Overpopulation in India – Causes, Effects and How to Control it?. Publication: 31.07.14. (Withdrawal from the internet: 08.04.16)

- http://www.mkgandhi.org/articles/g_health.htm. Mittal Chauhan: Gandhian Views on Health. (Withdrawal from the internet: 01.05.16)

- http://www.patengemeinschaft.de/seiten/indien/land.html. Patengemeinschaft für hungernde Kinder e.V.: Land und Leute. (Withdrawal from the Internet: 08.04.16)

- http://www.poverties.org/poverty-in-india.html. Poverties: Effects of Poverty in India: Between Injustice and Exclusion. Publication: 07.2011. (Withdrawal from the internet: 10.04.16)

- http://www.rsby.gov.in/about_rsby.aspx. RSBY: About RSBY. (Withdrawal from the internet: 24.04.16)

- http://www.skeptic.com/eskeptic/13-10-09/#note12. Marc Carrier: Ayurvedic Medicine It's been around for a thousand years, but does it work?. (Withdrawal from the internet: 17.04.16)

- http://www.thenational.ae/business/economy/indians-faced-with-overcrowded-public-hospitals-turn-to-private-clinics#full. Rebecca Bundhun: Indians faced with overcrowded public hospitals turn to private clinics. Publication: 22.09.14. (Withdrawal from the internet: 08.04.16)

- http://www.vsfs.cz/prilohy/konference/1_ws_3_1_theodopulos.doc. Sotiris Theodoropoulos: On the effectiveness of Publicly or Privately produced Health care services. (Withdrawal from the internet: 08.04.16)

- http://www.welt.de/gesundheit/article116481982/Klinik-bietet-Herz-Operationen-fuer-1390-Euro-an.html. Welt: Klinik bietet Herz-Operationen für 1390 Euro an. Publication: 24.05.13. (Withdrawal from the internet: 10.04.16)

- https://de.wikipedia.org/wiki/Berlin. Wikipedia: Berlin. (Withdrawal from the internet: 07.05.16)

- https://de.wikipedia.org/wiki/Gesetzliche_Unfallversicherung_in_Deutschland. Wikipedia: Gesetzliche Unfallversicherung in Deutschland. (Withdrawal from the internet: 07.05.16)

- https://de.wikipedia.org/wiki/Mumbai. Wikipedia: Mumbai. (Withdrawal from the internet: 07.05.16)

- https://en.wikipedia.org/wiki/Demographics_of_India. Wikipedia: Demographics of India. (Withdrawal from the internet: 1.05.16)

- https://en.wikipedia.org/wiki/Healthcare_in_Germany. Wikipedia: Healthcare in Germany. (Withdrawal from the internet: 07.05.16)

- https://en.wikipedia.org/wiki/Healthcare_in_India. Wikipedia: Healthcare in India. (Withdrawal from the internet: 01.05.16)

- https://en.wikipedia.org/wiki/Long-term_care_insurance_in_Germany. Wikipedia: Long-term care insurance in Germany. (Withdrawal from the internet: 07.05.16)

- https://en.wikipedia.org/wiki/Rashtriya_Swasthya_Bima_Yojana. Wikipedia: Rashtriya Swasthya Bima Yojana. (Withdrawal from the internet: 24.04.16)

- https://mygov.in/sites/default/files/user_comments/Current_Health.pdf. Ashok Vikhe Patil: Current Health Scenario In Rural India. Publication: 2012. (Withdrawal from the internet: 17.04.16)

- https://www.fmglobal-touchpoints.de/risiken-nutzen/laenderreport-indien/. FM Global: Länderreport Indien: Infrastrukturprobleme und Regierungsmaßnahmen. Publication: 21.08.15. (Withdrawal from the internet: 06.05.17)

- https://www.fondationalphabetisation.org/en/foundation/causes-of-illiteracy/consequences-of-illiteracy/. Literacy foundation: Consequences of illiteracy. (Withdrawal from the internet: 17.04.16)

- https://www.gesundheitsinformation.de/das-deutsche-gesundheitssystem.2698.de.html?part=einleitung-co. Institut für Qualität und Wirtschaftlichkeit im Gesundheitswesen: Das deutsche Gesundheitssystem. (Withdrawal from the internet: 07.05.16)

- https://www.giz.de/de/downloads/giz2013-de-akzente01-krankenversicherungsprogramm-indien.pdf. Rolph Schmachtenberg, GIZ: Eintrittskarte ins Sozialsystem. (Withdrawal from the internet: 24.04.16)

- https://www.justlanded.com/deutsch/Deutschland/Artikel/Gesundheit/Die-2-Arten-der-Krankenversicherung. Antonia Wolschon: Die zwei Arten der Krankenversicherung: Unterschied zwischen gesetzlicher und privater Versicherung. (Withdrawal from the internet: 07.05.16)

- https://www.private-krankenversicherungen-testsieger.de/private-krankenversicherung-vorteile-und-nachteile/. PKVT: Private Krankenversicherung Vorteile und Nachteile. (Withdrawal from the internet: 07.05.16)

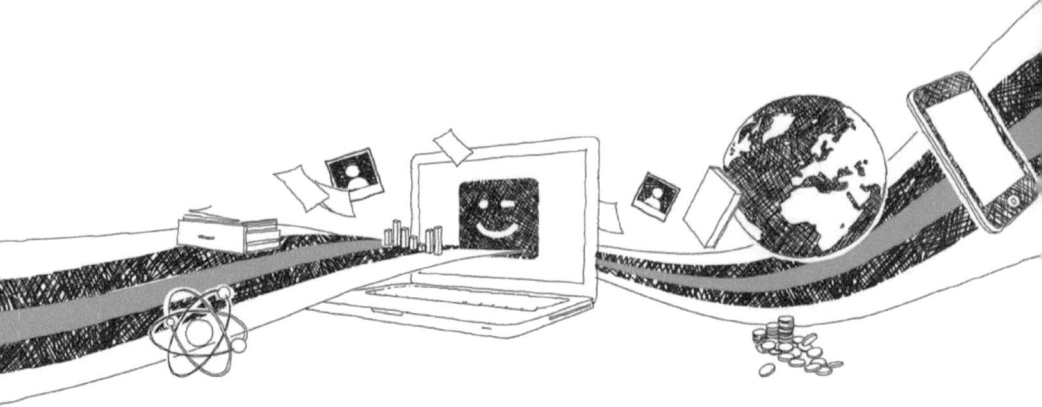
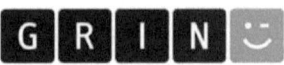